THE CANNABIS AND PHARMACY

GROW CANNABIS, MAKE HEMP OIL AND KNOW THE DIFFERENCE BETWEEN THC, CBD AND THE MEDICAL BENEFITS OF CANNABINOIDS

BY SMART READS

I0478373

Free Audiobook

As a thank you for being a Smart Reader you can choose 2 FREE audiobooks from audible.com. Simply sign up for free by visiting www.audibletrial.com/Travis to get your books.

Visit:
www.smartreads.co/freebooks
to receive Smart Reads books for FREE

Check us out on Instagram:
www.instagram.com/smart_readers
@smart_readers

ABOUT SMARTREADS

Choose Smart Reads and get smart every time. Smart Reads sorts through all the best content and condenses the most helpful information into easily digestible chunks.

We design our books to be short, easy to read and highly informative. Leaving you with maximum understanding in the least amount of time.

Smart Reads aims to accelerate the spread of quality information so we've taken the copyright off everything we publish and donate our material directly to the public domain. You can read our uncopyright below.

We believe in paying it forward and donate 5% of our net sales to Pencils of Promise to build schools, train teachers and support child education.

To limit our footprint and restore forests around the globe we are planting a tree for every 10 hardcover books we sell.

Thanks for choosing Smart Reads and helping us help the planet.

Sincerely,

Travis & the Smart Reads Team

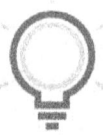

TABLE OF CONTENTS

INTRODUCTION

Cannabis, also known as marijuana (and other names), is a genus of flowering plant belonging to the Cannabaceae family. Cannabis plants can be grown worldwide and are found nearly everywhere today. It is indigenous to central Asia and the Indian subcontinent, and is thought to have originated in the mountainous areas of the Himalayas.

The cannabis plant flower annually with the first leaves appearing to have only a single leaflet. The most leaflets that can be on a leaf are thirteen per leaf but the average is usually seven to nine. The flowers of the cannabis plant are usually imperfect and contain either "male" or "female" flowers, with some plants bearing both.

Cannabis plants produce chemicals known as cannabinoids. These are the chemicals that produce both mental and physical effects when they are consumed. As a drug, cannabis is usually available in dried flower buds known as marijuana, or resin, also known as hashish. Cannabis has been a banned plant and drug in most parts of the world for the past century. However, today it is making a comeback and its medicinal qualities are beginning to be recognized by the scientific and medical professions.

Many people have experienced amazing pain relief by using CBD and medical marijuana. It is likely that CBD and medical marijuana will continue to change the medical arena and that legislation and legalization will make it more available to greater numbers of people who can benefit from the medical qualities it possesses.

This book is intended to share information about CBD or cannabidiol - the cannabis compound that has some significant medical benefits. You'll learn what cannabinoids can do to the brain and the body, and the way in which they are beneficial, even becoming a great alternative to most medicines.

This book is intended to be easily readable, however, there is some technical language used with descriptions in order to give you clearer information about cannabis and its uses.

IMPORTANT NOTE:

This book is intended to provide reliable information and is as exact as possible at the time of writing. It is in no way intended to replace the advice of a physician and readers are encouraged to check with a doctor if they have any type of health concerns.

If you have serious conditions such as cancer, epilepsy, COPD or any other serious disease or condition where both CBD and also THC may have some medical potential, it is necessary for you to discuss this in detail with a medical practitioner and find out how CBD might interact with any medication you might be taking to prevent potential side effects which may be harmful.

Below is only a short list of drugs that will interact with the Cannabidiol. It contains drugs that are metabolized by cytochrome P-450, which your doctor will also know about. The below information comes from the Indiana University Department of Medicine. It includes, but is not necessarily limited to:

- HMG CoA reductase inhibitors
- Steroids
- Antihistamines
- Prokinetics

- Calcium channel blockers
- HIV antivirals
- Benzodiazepines
- Immune modulators
- Antibiotics
- Anti-arrythmics
- Anti-psychotics
- Anesthetics
- Anti-epileptics
- Anti-depressants
- PPIs
- Beta blockers
- Angiotension II blockers
- NSAIDs
- Sulfonylureas Oral hypoglycemic agents

Please remember that the list above does not contain every type of medication that might be affected by the use of cannabidiol. It is also necessary to note that not all the medications listed above will actually cause any type of interaction. This is why you must always consult a doctor before taking any combination of drugs. Dosage adjustments or in some cases alternate medications may be needed. For those who might be worried that their P-450 enzyme system isn't working properly, your doctor can check this for you to ensure the medications taken are metabolizing correctly.

It's also worth remembering that not all doctors or medical professionals will be aware of or even in favor of medical cannabis due to it being a new concept and also because of a bias on behalf of the medical practitioner involved. However, in such a situation it is best if you can find a medical professional who has knowledge of this subject and can provide you with some sound medical advice. Also, please check the legality of using medical cannabis in your state or country.

This book is intended to provide information to readers and to focus on the more important effects CBD can have, while ensuring it is easily digestible. As mentioned earlier, be aware that the medical use of cannabis and CBD could have some unwanted and/or detrimental side effects when used with certain pharmaceutical drugs. If that might be the case for you, it's worth stressing again that professional advice from a trained medical expert must be sought.

CHAPTER 1: WHAT IS CBD?

Before we begin, it is important for you to know terms like THC and CBD and what they stand for. THC is short for Tetrahydrocannabinol and is the compound found in certain cannabis plants that have a psychoactive effect on the brain. It is what gives people the "high" when the plant is smoked or taken orally (as in food).

CBD is short for cannabidiol, a compound found in the well-known and once illicit cannabis as well as the legal industrial component of cannabis, which is called hemp. It now seems like CBD has quite a lot to offer. The CBD compound has significant medical benefits without getting "high" part of it. It was only in recent years that cannabis, CBD and THC, have seen positive media attention and this attention has removed the stigma of it being an illegal Schedule I drug. Marijuana legalization has become a hot topic in the last few years, especially as twenty-nine states in the U.S. approved the use of medical marijuana. In eight different states, recreational marijuana usage has also been approved.

This legal status is not only limited to the U.S. The U.K. also has laws allowing limited use of medical cannabis, and Canadians have been able to use it for medical purposes since June 2015. In many European countries, marijuana is often illegal but decriminalized, and in places such as Australia, Cambodia, India, and Uruguay, the least restrictive cannabis laws exist. In Australia, some states have legalized the use of medical marijuana from 2016.

Since cannabis is being used legally more and more today, a large amount of information is available to consider. People need to know what CBD is. You should also know the differences between CBD and THC, as mentioned above. In addition, you will need to have information on how CBD works and its possible effects on the body and the brain. CBD will be further explained in this chapter.

As mentioned above, CBD is in reference to cannabidiol; it is the short version of the word. It is a cannabinoid from the cannabis plant or hemp and is 1 of at least 115 active cannabinoids that have been identified in the cannabis plant. Cannabinoids exists in two cannabis species: 1.) cannabis sativa and 2.) cannabis indica. Hemp is a part of the cannabis sativa family and there is a big difference in the CBD/THC levels for industrial cannabis and also the cannabis drug or cannabis medicine.

Over the past few years, cannabis has been planted and grown for its levels of THC and also its CBD; however, hemp has remained the same due to the plant materials needed for industrial production. For this reason, big changes in cannabinoid containment and the CBD and THC levels are much lower.

THC is the main psychoactive compound in cannabis. Cannabidiol, on the other hand, comes in second place. CBD accounts for around 40% of cannabis' extract. However, different strains of cannabis will contain different levels of both compounds.

CBD is also a non-psychoactive compound. It was discovered in the year 1940; however, its chemical structure and its stereochemistry were identified in 1964, more than 20 years later.

Today, more and more information is coming out about what CBD can do and the studies are showing potentially positive effects. At this point negative effects of CBD remain at zero. More recent studies show this compound has immense medicinal benefits instead.

It is CBD, (cannabidiol) which is today changing the debate surrounding medical marijuana usage. The focus has now shifted from THC in cannabis, which would get people high, to the other compound, CBD, and for very good reason. CBD doesn't seem to have any side effects and doctors and researchers are beginning to seriously look at what medical benefits it contains.

Five Important Facts About CBD You Should Know

1. **CBD is a key ingredient found in cannabis -** Researchers have identified numerous compounds in cannabis. They belong to a group of molecules referred to as cannabinoids. CBD and also THC are generally found in higher concentrations, and for this reason they're being studied more often.

Different cannabis plants will have different levels of CBD and THC. For example, marijuana specifically grown for recreational purposes will contain more THC than it does CBD. By using certain breeding techniques, however, cannabis breeders have now created cannabis varieties with higher levels of CBD and close to zero levels of THC. These have become a lot more popular recently.

2. **CBD has no psychoactive properties** – CBD doesn't get people high and therefore has a significant advantage as medicine. Health professionals and patients prefer a treatment that will have minimal side

effects. Of course, this makes high CBD cannabis a poor choice for recreational users of marijuana.

In 2011, a review published in Current Drug Safety, found that CBD doesn't interfere with many psychological and psychomotor functions. They mentioned that CBD is "well tolerated and safe" even when administered at higher doses.

3. **CBD has many medicinal benefits** – In 2013, a review was published in the British Journal of Clinical Pharmacology, which stated that CBD was found to have numerous medical properties. These include:

- Anticonvulsant – suppresses seizure activity
- Anti-inflammatory – Fights inflammatory disorders
- Antiemetic – reduces vomiting and nausea
- Anti-oxidant – Fights neurodegenerative illnesses
- Antipsychotic – Combats many psychosis disorders
- Anti-cancer/anti-tumoral – Fights cancer and tumor cells
- Anti-depressant – Fights depression and anxiety

Much of this information was derived from animal studies but more and more research is being done on humans. A UK company is already funding clinical trials of CBD as treatment for epilepsy and schizophrenia. At the California Pacific Medical Center, Dr. McAllister has said they would like to start trials on CBD as a therapy for breast cancer.

4. **CBD can reduce negative effects of THC** – CBD at this point, seems to be a natural protector against the "high" that marijuana produces. Many studies have suggested that CBD reduces any intoxicating effects of THC like paranoia and memory impairment, and its sleep inducing effects. Neither CBD nor THC poses any risk of lethal overdose, however, in order to reduce any side effects the cannabis with high CBD levels should be used.

5. **In many parts of the world, CBD is still illegal** – CBD has shown a lot of medicinal promise but is still illegal in many countries. It is still considered a Schedule 1 drug in the U.S. and Canada, however, as mentioned before, many states are now allowing medical cannabis to be used and in some U.S. states, recreational marijuana has been decriminalized.

Despite the fact it is still classified as a Schedule 1 drug, the U.S. Food and Drug Administration has approved a trial for a pharmaceutical CBD version for children with some rare types of epilepsy. The company states that the drug consists of 98% CBD and zero THC levels. The other two percent is made up of other cannabinoids.

How Do Cannabinoids Work?

Phytocannabinoids, like both CBD and THC, are a diverse chemical compound class found in the cannabis plant and hemp that act on the cannabinoid receptors found in body cells. They change neurotransmitter releases in the brain like THC changes dopamine release, the neurotransmitter is also referred to as the "feel good" chemical.

Within the brain there are several cannabinoid receptors. These are known as being part of the endocannabinoid system. Two of the receptors are now defined as CB1 and CB2. Two of these cannabinoid receptors are also common in animals. They are found in fish, birds, reptiles, and mammals.

Cannabinoid Receptors Type 1 or CB1

CB1, are receptors found mostly in the human brain, or more specifically, they are found in the basal nuclei as well as in the limbic system, including the hippocampus. CB1 is also found in the part of the brain that regulates and co-ordinates muscular activity, the cerebellum. It is also in the female and the male reproductive systems. This accounts for certain effects once THC, as an example, changes the neurotransmitter release of dopamine from the cannabinoid receptors that are in the brain.

Cannabinoid Receptors Type 2 or CB2
CB2's are mostly found in the immune cells or the immune system. The highest concentration of which is found in the spleen. They are found in what is the outlying nervous system that runs throughout the body in order to connect the limbs and the organs to the body's central nervous system located in the spinal cord and the brain. Its job is to act as a communication line between the brain and the spinal cord with the rest of the body. The CB2 receptors appear to be in charge of any anti-inflammatory properties and other possible therapeutic benefits of cannabis.

CHAPTER 2: CDB – WHAT DOES IT DO?

As mentioned, different cannabis plants will have differing levels of CBD and THC. For example, marijuana specifically grown for recreational purposes will contain more THC than it does CBD. By using certain breeding techniques, cannabis breeders have created cannabis varieties with higher levels of CBD and close to zero levels of THC. This kind of marijuana is more popular today because CBD has no psychoactive properties. CBD doesn't get people high so it's uses as medicine is much more significant.

CBD doesn't interfere with bodily functions, both physical and psychological. And even when administered in high doses, it's still found to be considerably safe.

Cannabidiol counteracts the cognitive impairment associated with cannabis usage. It is non-psychotropic therefore it does not have an attraction to THC and certain other cannabinoid agonists, which are substances that initiate a physiological response when combined with receptors. What this means in plain language is that CBD will counteract any cognitive impairment people often associate with using cannabis. When you put all this information together you can conclude that CBD does indeed have some potential medically.

Cannabidiol also works on more receptors, not only CB1 and CB2. It mainly affects the receptors adenosine, serotonin, and vanilloid. The vallinoid receptor is responsible for detecting and regulating body temperature. It provides the sensations of pain and scolding heat and is also responsible for pain felt after eating hot peppers, for example, which make the body sweat. Cannabidiol mediates and therefore has shown itself to be an anti-inflammatory helping to lessen pain.

These functions are already impressive enough, however, they are not the only ones that CBD is responsible for inside the body. Through more recent studies it has been discovered how CBD works in stimulating the serotonin receptor, which is a known anti-depressant producer. This particular receptor is found in a wide range of processes including perception, appetite, anxiety, nausea, addiction mechanisms, and pain.

Moreover, CBD tends to decrease the expansion of cancer cells and enhances bone reabsorption by inhibiting the GPR55 signaling which has been linked to essential processes such as the control of blood pressure, the modulation of bone density, as well as prevention of the continued production of the cancerous cells. There will be some more information on this when we discuss CBD health benefits and how to use it as medicine a little further into the book.

Medical Usage and Medical Application
The most recent studies show that CBD has these medical properties:

- Antipsychotic (fights psychosis disorders)
- Antiemetic (combats vomiting and nausea)
- Anti-inflammatory
- Anticonvulsant (suppresses most seizure activity)
- Anti-cancerous/ anti-tumoral (combats cancer and tumor cells)
- Anti-depressant/ Anxiolytic (combats stress and anxiety disorders)
- Anti-oxidant (combats disorders of the neurodegenerative kind)

CBD as an Anti-Inflammatory
Many studies have recently reported that CBD shows neuroprotective properties within cell structures. Animal studies in models with a number of neurodegenerative diseases like multiple sclerosis, Alzheimer's, glutamine toxicity, Parkinson's disease,

and other neurodegenerative diseases such as brain damage that has been caused due to alcohol abuse, have been done and the results are promising.

Many recent studies and also clinic trails have shown that the medicine, which contains CBD properties, has been successful in treating spasticity that is associated with Multiple Sclerosis. It also lessened the severity of spasticity in patients with MS.

With regards to people with Parkinson's disease, CBD has some serious benefits to offer them. CBD has the ability to improve the complex sleep-behaviors associated with REM sleep (rapid eye movement) behavior disorders. It does this by rapidly reducing symptoms of this disorder and then helping with the improvement of sleep quality. This being the case, it's safe to suggest that CBD treatment has showed that this cannabinoid improved the quality-of-life elements significantly for those patients who suffer from the debilitating Parkinson's disease.

CBD as an Anticonvulsant
Over the last decade, studies have been conducted that show how cannabinoids work in creating an anti-seizure effect. The studies reported that cannabinoids reduce the seizures' severity in all animal models used. To make things even more interesting and

optimistic, case studies have been done on children and the CBD effects measured with those who suffer from epilepsy that is drug resistant. The results so far suggest enormous medicinal benefits through CBD usage.

CBD as Anti-Cancerous/Anti-Tumoral
Over the past few years several lines of evidence have supported the anti-cancerous/anti-tumoral effects of cannibinoids. CBD possesses anti-apoptotic and anti-proliferative properties that are known to interfere with tumor growth, cancer cell migration, invasion, adhesion, and metastasization. Patients with cancer who are being treated with CBD are showing positive results and the trials are continuing.

CBD helps patients maintain a proper appetite just for starters. It also helps to reduce pain and offset sleeping problems. It is thought that these CBD abilities are because of the anti-inflammatory and anti-oxidant qualities it possesses.

Considering medical cannabis has shown such enormous success and even more potential in the treatment of human cancer patients, it's clear CBD should now get more acknowledgement from the medical world so that it can be prioritized and people can start getting the best of whatever CBD has to offer humans.

CBD as Stress Reliever and Anti-Psychotic
Most people know that cannabis does indeed have the potential to set off severe psychotic episodes when taken at higher doses and under specific circumstances. There have been several studies that have linked marijuana usage to increased risks of chronic psychosis for some individuals who have specific risk factors of a genetic nature. The research conducted in a few studies and also some clinical trials suggest it is the THC that has mediated those effects. It has also been proposed that it is CBD that counteracts psychotic episodes and works as an actual anti-psychotic. Furthermore, it is able to alleviate the effects or the THC.

Over the past few years there have also been a number of clinical trials on a smaller-scale where patients who presented with psychotic symptoms have been treated with the CBD cannabis. This includes reports of some patients suffering from schizophrenia.

There have been conflicting results there. In one smaller case study whereby patients who have Parkinson's disease and psychosis were administered CBD, positive results were reported after their treatment with CBD. In another small and random clinical trial, patients who suffer from schizophrenia were reported to have shown improvement after taking CBD for a period of time.

Considering all the information gained from the smaller scale trials, it is easy to see that the potential is definitely there and that larger random clinical trials are needed in order to fully evaluate CBD's therapeutic potential. These trials will focus on certain illnesses including schizophrenia, bipolar, and certain other types of psychosis.

Through studies already conducted, CBD has shown it is able to reduce stress and anxiety. This, in turn, reduces behavioral issues as well as physiological ones like increased heart rate, for example, when it was tested on animal models. Some smaller clinical and laboratory trials were done using human models and the results were positive indeed. Reports from those trials showed that CBD reduces anxiety and stress in patients who had social anxiety. The patients were tested while doing a high-stress public speaking type task.

There has also been a laboratory study which was created to model PTSD or post- traumatic stress disorder. It was found that CBD enhanced "consolidation of extinction learning," which means it has the ability to help patients forget some traumatic memories. CBD's anxiety-reducing benefits seem to be activated or triggered by changing the serotonin receptor 1 signaling. More research needs to be done, however, to better and more fully understand the way it works.

CHAPTER 3: APPLICATIONS OF CBD

Now that you've got information and understanding on CBD, what it is, its effects and benefits and how it works on several conditions using research and laboratory reporting, it's best to understand the way CBD products are made and also applied in daily life.

For starters, CBD hemp oil or hempseed oil is the most common CBD form. This is taken solely from the seeds and therefore it does not contain any THC, or the properties that create the "high." CBD does, however, have other different applications. These include edibles, tinctures, topicals, and pure concentrates. These come in pure CBD live resin that comes directly from the cannabis plant and made into special types of edible products like chocolate bars and ointment creams. These products can be bought throughout Europe and the U.S. in homeopathic pharmacies, online stores, dispensaries and also as prescription drugs through a health professional's medical advice, the last one of course, depends on the country or state in which you live.

Medical cannabis is a personalized type of medicine. The correct regimen and dosage is needed and it all depends on the individual person and on his/her condition. It is important that the right amount is used in order to achieve the maximum therapeutic benefits. One of the key factors in determining the correct CBD medicine dosage is your own personal sensitivity. There are some products available which contain both CBD and THC and some people might not find THC pleasant.

The correct balance between both levels must be worked out if this is the case, in order to get more effective treatment. As mentioned in the Important Notes section, it is imperative for you to get advice from a medical professional.

For people who suffer from anxiety, depression, spasms, or pediatric seizures, sometimes the best kind of treatment can be found in a moderate dosage of a product that is CBD dominant with a ratio of 10:1 of CBD/THC. However, treating these conditions or illnesses with a particular product which has even a low THC level isn't always the most effective or best option, despite it not being intoxicating. In some cases, people will get better effects using a combination (for some conditions) than THC or CBD alone.

For certain conditions such as neurological diseases, cancer, and various other illnesses, some patients could benefit from using a balanced ratio of THC and CBD. Vast clinical research has been conducted and shows that a 1:1 THC/CBD ratio can be very effective indeed for those suffering from neuropathic pain. If you decide to optimize your medicinal use of cannabis you must make sure it is approached step by step.

It is a process whereby you must attempt to get the best balance possible of the CBD/THC ratio in the medicinal dosage and one that matches the condition or illness you are treating. This provides you with an opportunity to begin with smaller doses of non-intoxicating cannabis products rich in CBD. Watch and assess the results you get then you can decide to gradually increase the amounts and perhaps use a mixture of CBD and small amounts of THC. It's worth mentioning again, a doctor's advice is best and self-medication of any type of drug can be dangerous.

CBD Oil and How to Use It
CBD oil brands have different consumption standards and different dosing; therefore consumers tend to become confused. In many cases, these brands will recommend either too much as a dosage or "serving" or they will recommend not enough. The average would be around 25mg of CBD to be taken twice a day.

Again it must be stressed that a health professional should be consulted and this book is to be only used as a guide. Please refer any questions to your doctor.

Some people might be able to increase the dosage by 25 mgs. every 3 or 4 weeks. This can be done until they get relief from their symptoms. If it is clear that the symptoms are becoming worse then, the CBD amount must be lessened. The CBD oil concentrations, the extracts and the concentrates can vary between the preparations for medicinal use. This could range from 1 mg. per dose up to hundreds of milligrams. Due to this it can be easier to get the needed dosages in a particular form that is easier to use for the individual that is taking it.

For the treatment of chronic pain: 2.5-20 mg of CBD orally. This is to be taken an average of about 25 days.

For increasing the appetite of cancer patients: 2.5 milligrams of THC taken orally. This can be taken with or without the 1 mg of CBD for around six weeks.

For the treatment of epilepsy: 200-300 mg CBD to be taken orally every day for up to 4 ½ months.

For the treatment of sleep disorders: 40-160 mg CBD to be taken orally.

For the treatment of movement difficulties linked to Huntington's disease (for this you will need to know body weight): 10 mg of CBD for each kilogram of bodyweight. It is to be taken orally every day for 6 weeks.

For the treatment of schizophrenia: 40-1,280 mg of CBD orally every day for up to four weeks.

For the treatment of multiple sclerosis symptoms: Take cannabis plant extracts that contain 2.5-120 milligrams of THC and CBD combinations. This is to be taken orally every day for 2 to 15 weeks. Mouth sprays can be used and might contain about 2.5 milligrams of CBD and 2.7 milligrams of THC at doses of 2.5-120 milligrams. This should be done for up to 8 weeks. The typical usage is 8 sprays within any three-hour period. The maximum spray dosage is 48 sprays within a 24-hour period.

For the treatment of glaucoma: one dosage of 20-40 mg CBD placed under the tongue. Be careful here as a dose of more than 40mg might increase eye pressure.

No established dose of lethal CBD exists right now, but reading product inserts carefully is imperative to make sure the correct CBD amount is being taken. Also make sure you talk to a medical practitioner regarding any concerns or questions you may have.

CHAPTER 4: CANNABIS GROWING ENVIRONMENTS

In today's world, growing plants in a controlled environment is a modern farming technique. It is a great way to optimize limited space as well as crop yield. Cannabis grown in controlled environments provide several advantages, the biggest one being that the crops can be managed to produce lifecycles and quality. The plants can be produced the same in every way due to the fact that the grow room is a simulated environment and every plant is the same. Grow rooms are indoors and are often enclosed spaces which are sterile and devoted solely to growing the cannabis plant.

In grow rooms, another advantage is disease control. If, for any reason, there is an outbreak of a disease, it can be kept to a minimum and then eliminated. The infected plant can be easily identified and destroyed, thereby lessening the chance of anything spreading.

Cannabis farmers try to recreate all natural environment elements. Many choices exist for choosing growing mediums for the cannabis plant. Many growers use potting soil or a soil-less mix. Fertilizers are also used unless the grower is using soil-less mixes that have adequate amounts to grow cannabis. Some chemical fertilizers are commonly used because they contain Nitrogen, Phosphorous and Potassium, things the cannabis plant thrives on.

Proper lighting is also necessary and it must always be regulated correctly when growing indoor cannabis. Fluorescent lights can be used for seedlings and clones, but for plants that have grown a higher intensity (HID) lighting is needed. This will help the plants grow into the vegetative and flowering stages.

Grow rooms need specific wiring for their electricity usage. In the rooms there will be lights, perhaps timers, and fans, all of which need electrical powering. Due to the lights being a higher wattage in grow rooms, a different circuit is necessary and not just the regular one found in an average house.

A lot of water is needed to grow cannabis. The water must be good quality but tap water can be used as long as it is safe for drinking. Proper drainage channels are also necessary in grow rooms for the excess water to flow through.

CHAPTER 5: HOW CAN CBD HEMP OIL BE USED TO MAKE CBD PRODUCTS?

Farms, gardens, and companies that cultivate cannabis to produce CBD hemp oil will have seasonal harvests that yield high CBD and low THC cannabis strains. The harvested buds and other plant materials will then be put through a specialized extradition process, which is solvent-free.

In this way the hemp oil has a very high cannabidiol concentration and it remains purer. The pure hemp extract must then be tested for its quality, its safety, and also the cannibidiol content before it is processed and made into CBD products or before they are placed on shelves in stores to be sold directly as concentrates.

In the U.S. where cannabis is not legal in some states, when it comes to cannabis products their medical use can be somewhat restricted. In this case importing may be the only choice because CBD is legal. However, you will need to get the industrial grade hemp should you decide to make this yourself.

This can, unfortunately, make CBD expensive in the U.S. where importing may be the only course for some to take, depending on which state they live in.

Making CBD Cannabis Oil Yourself

Important note: It is absolutely imperative that anyone considering using the method explained in this book to extract CBD read the following. Since you will be using alcohol as the solvent, it is necessary and of utmost importance that you remain vigilant of the surroundings, in particular concerning any stoves, open fires, smoking and any other situations that might create potential harm or if there is a risk of anything catching fire.

Before Starting - Measuring Your CBD Containments

If you want the safest and most precise way to test how many milligrams of CBD your CBD extract actually contains, it will be necessary to take it to a lab and have it tested. Of course, this isn't always an affordable or available option. If this is the case, there is a little trick that you should know if you are measuring it yourself. This particular method of measuring the CBD is not the most accurate; however, it will assist you in getting an idea of the dosage and purity within your plant material.

One recommendation is to only use the buds that are consumer-standard grown medical cannabis and are not for recreational use. You can get these from certified farms and dispensaries. This would mean that you are getting the buds that have already been lab tested for their CBD/THC levels. This would also mean you know exactly what percentage of THC and CBD the cannabis you are buying contains in each gram.

If you are free to choose which strain you want, and there may be several that you can choose from that have already been tested for CBD and THC levels, it would be better to choose the cannabis strains that have higher concentrations of CBD and lower concentrations of THC in order to get the best CBD oil extractions.

An important thing to know, for those of you who are very new to all of this, is that, the THC levels are very different from CBD levels. A 1-5% of THC is considered a low THC level, whereas 1-5% of CBD is quite high for a cannabis strain. Therefore, if you are looking at the highest end of a THC strain, you should have 15-25% THC per gram. For the CBD levels, you should be looking at 14-15% for the highest CBD strain cannabis. The differing compound amounts in cannabis plants are a major aspect of creating newer medical marijuana strains to grow buds that have higher levels of THC and CBD.

The thing you should ultimately be looking for in a good quality CBD extract is 1.) a good CBD strain which has already been tested and known to have high CBD levels that range from 5-15%, and 2.) the THC levels remain at 5% or preferably even less. If it is legal in your area and you decide to grow some marijuana yourself, the CBD/THC levels should already be provided for you with the seeds. This is why it is important that you buy your seeds from reputable and professional cannabis seed companies.

Those companies will be able to offer a large variety of seeds that are high in CBD and low in THC. You will then be able to choose seeds that are a good fit for your medical marijuana needs. For example, if you need a particular balance of compounds such as high THC and low CBD oil for daily usage, you can get this. It will provide you with the energizing and uplifting effects of the THC and the levels of CBD you need.

What it all boils down to is this - 1% of a single gram equals 10 milligrams. Therefore, if what you have is a strain which contains 2% CBD and 15% THC it will contain 20 milligrams of CBD and 150 milligrams of THC. This is how you can measure the cannabis buds you're using if they've been lab-tested and have the CBD and THC levels provided. If you do not have seeds from a reputable company or have not grown the marijuana yourself then there really is not much you can do if the levels of CBD and THC are not what you would have preferred.

It is possible to estimate the CBD and THC levels in the cannabis going by the effect it has. As is well known, a strain which contains higher THC and lower or no CBD levels will give the person an energizing, uplifting feeling. It will tend to be positive but may also make you feel a little anxious. If you purchase unfamiliar strains or even cannabis that is bought illegally and has higher levels of CBD of around 5% per gram, it can still get you stoned or high. These particular strains will help you relax, sedating you and counteract anxiety and stress.

It is impossible you will ever get a pure strain of CBD cannabis on the street as a recreational drug. This is because the effects of the pure CBD cannabis are very much medical and will not get people high. The strains of 5 to 15% CBD and low THC will not get people stoned or high because CBD will counter the psychoactive effect of the small THC amount in that strain. If you are looking for these then the only places you should be looking at are local dispensaries or you could consider growing them yourself.

It is never recommended that you buy marijuana illegally. Apart from the fact it is illegal, it also has not been tested and this type of cannabis also has the risk of containing powders like milk powder, calcium or other materials, even pesticides. They do this to add weight and of course, charge people more. In some cases, it could be possible that glossy, glasslike chemicals like hairspray or glass powder have actually been used in order to make it seem like a bud that is densely covered in THC.

If you buy illegally you also run the risk that the illegally purchased and most likely untested cannabis has been contaminated with angel dust (PCP). This is a dissociative drug and can bring on hallucinations and violent episodes. Illegally bought cannabis might also have other chemical drugs and these are used to improve its effects. It is dangerous and this is not recommended at all.

The way these cannabis strains have been added to has nothing to do with the actual plant itself. It is just a dark side of the drug trade and why there is another urgent and important reason for cannabis to be legalized. You must remember that this particular component of the cannabis business is illegal and it usually does not have any thought or concern for the people using it because there is a lot of money involved.

How to Measure Cannabis Oil Containments
It is here that things get a bit harder regarding how to measure your own cannabis oil. If you can go to a lab and get the oil tested it is highly recommended that you do so because the method mentioned below isn't always accurate. If you have a larger amount of oil and of used cannabis it will be easier to measure CBD and THC levels as long as you have correct information. You will have to use the same formula for calculating the CBD. It is easier to weigh the amounts when they're in larger quantities.

To give you an example, let's say you have 453 grams (or 1 pound) of cannabis buds that are lab tested and they have 15.9% CBD and 9.5% THC, there would be 43,035 grams of THC. There is 95miligrams of THC in one gram therefore if you calculate 95 x 453 : 1000 = 43,035 grams of THC in pounds). Now the same formula would apply for calculating how much CBD is present. What you do is calculate the 159 mg of CBD, which is in a gram, and multiply it by how much cannabis you have – 453 grams – then divide whatever the outcome is through 1000 and you should have 72,027 grams of CBD in one pound of cannabis buds. This would be if they were tested at 15.9% CBD and 9.5% THC. Knowing this should ensure you can potentially have a 100% pure return in cannabis oil and it should be 114,052 grams.

The above is basically a perfect extraction and almost impossible to do without having the proper knowledge and experience.

Cheesecloth will be used to extract and strain the material of the plant and the raw buds to make the oil. This will mean you'll have the residue of the plant left over in the oil that will then bring down the concentration level. However, people have made some good homemade oils (that have been tested) going by this particular method. When lab tested it was found to have 70-95% purity.

Now you have more of an idea what you're looking for if you decide to make cannabis oil on your own and you want to, as accurately as possible, measure the CBD and THC amounts. It is better if it can be as accurate as possible, of course. To give an example, let's say you have had your oil tested and it is found to be 85% pure oil with 35% THC and 50% CBD content in every 100 grams.

This would then mean you've got around 15 grams plant residue in the oil and the oil is of high quality and potent. For those who know their math and can calculate using the metric system, it will be easy to do the calculations provided that you have all the correct information regarding the type of cannabis you are using.

CHAPTER 6: MAKING CBD OIL

Below are the instructions on how to process grain alcohol extraction of cannabis oil. This particular process will get you around 2 to 4 grams of very high potency, medicinal-grade CBD oil and it is fine to be ingested. Once you have done a couple of practice runs it will probably take you around an hour to make a small batch of ingestible oil. This includes the 30 minutes that it takes to cook. Using grain alcohol for this process is best because it is the ingredient least likely to leave residue or impurities in your final product.

What you will need:
• 1 ounce dried and ground bud material
• 2-3 ounces ground and dried trim shake
• 1 gallon solvent – this would be the grain alcohol or another higher proof alcohol). **Never use any sort of rubbing alcohol.
• A mixing bowl of medium size (a glass bowl is preferred but ceramic is fine too)
• A catchment container
• A strainer. This could be cheesecloth, grain-steeping bags, muslin bags, clean nylon stockings, or a stainless steel sieve combo.
• A Baine Marie or double boiler
• A wooden spoon (large)

• A plastic syringe – this is for dispensing the oil and for dosage
• A funnel
• A silicon spatula

Process

1. Prepare the space you will work in (make sure it is level and clean) - arrange the necessary equipment.

2. Next, put the ground cannabis ingredients into your mixing bowl and ensure there is space left for the solvent. If you think there will not be enough room just get yourself a lager bowl.

3. Cover your plant material completely with alcohol. Add about one extra inch or so of solvent (alcohol) above the upper level of the plant matter into the bowl.

4. With your wooden spoon, stir the cannabis that's in the alcohol for approximately 3 minutes. This will enable the resin glands to better dissolve within the solvent. Ensure that all plant matter is totally saturated and that the resin content can be flushed out from the mixture.

5. Now place the sieve or straining bag into your catchment container and pour all the darkish green

liquid into the sieve or bag. Next step is to allow this liquid to completely filter then pour it into the catchment container. You will have to massage your bag gently (if that's what you're using) so you can squeeze as much liquid out as you possibly can.

Note: You can repeat the abovementioned four steps if you choose to do so to try and get even more resin extracted and into the solvent. It is this second "wash' that should then remove most of the resin that has remained.

6. When this is done pour the liquid that has been strained into the cooking pots or a double boiler, as with the Bain Marie where you place a small cooking pot into a larger one and place water in the pot at the bottom. Make sure there is enough water, but not too much. This will prevent the pot on top from cooking too quickly or from overheating. This might need to be done in batches if the alcohol-resin mixture doesn't all fit into the top part of the cooking pot or double boiler. You can just continue to refill the pot once the CBD oil is boiled down or until you have eventually processed all the rinse liquid.

7. Turn up the heat to high and put your double boiler onto it, heating until all the liquid inside it starts to bubble. This will be the alcohol that is evaporating. As

it is bubbling you can then turn the burner off. The heat that still remains in the water will continue to heat the mixture and allow the alcohol to continue evaporating.

8. If you see that the mixture has stopped bubbling, you might need to turn on the heat again perhaps one or two more times. This evaporation step of the process will take around 15-20 minutes to fully complete.

**Note: Throughout the process of evaporation this mixture should continue to bubble. The amount of bubbles will decrease as the levels of alcohol decrease. It's a good idea to mix the solution occasionally with a silicon spatula. Scrape the pan sides as you are mixing to make sure everything is mixed together and you get all of the mixture not just some.

9. Don't allow your mixture to become too hot. If this happens the cannabinoids will be damaged and of course, the potency and the flavor will then be compromised. Once your mixture isn't bubbling anymore but is still runny, put the heat level back to low. This will encourage the mixture to start bubbling once again. Once it does, turn the heat off. Continue stirring it as this will ensure even more of the alcohol is evaporated.

10. You will know when your oil is done once it is thick and has tar-like consistency. It should also not be bubbling anymore. The mixture will continue to get thicker as it cools down so you will now have to transfer your oil mixture into the dosage or storage containers.

11. Now you will have to draw the CBD oil slowly into plastic syringes. It will be a little more difficult once you've reached the pan bottom but this is quite normal. The remaining amounts can be transferred into some smaller containers that are airtight. You can squeeze out the smaller doses through the syringe but can also use a toothpick to portion off the dosages.

For those of you who prefer topical applications, all you need to do is combine CBD oil with some coconut or olive oil while it's still warm and hasn't cooled down. This will also decrease the potency as it will stretch the dosages out and can be a good idea for users who are less experienced or cash-strapped.

Process
1. Place oils into a ceramic, or preferably a glass-mixing bowl. If you're using a combination, you will have to use a wooden spoon and then mix them all well.

2. Place a large pot onto the stove filling it halfway (or a little less) with water.

3. Once the water has heated but isn't boiling, place the mixing bowl into the pot. Make sure no water at all gets in the bowl.

4. When all the oils are liquefied and they have blended well, add the cannabis.

5. At this point allow the mixture to gently simmer and stir every couple of minutes, for around 45 minutes. Hint: the longer the mixture can simmer the more potent the salve will be which is what we're looking for.

6. Now strain your salve through a cheesecloth and into a different glass container. Make sure to squeeze the cheesecloth so you can get every drop out from the cannabis mixture.

7. Let the mixture now completely cool before using it.

8. When it has cooled you could use a spatula or spoon to move the salve into another container.

9. Store it in a cool, dark place. This balm should keep for around two months.

* If you add beeswax to the oil it will help in making the (hand) balm a bit firmer and also more stable. If you use the beeswax alone you will have a hard substance. It can still be used for lip balm, however, if you do not want that, add one or more other oils into the mix.

*Both grape seed oil and almond oil are good for giving the mixture a smooth and non-greasy balm.

*For those of you who want a balm with a sweet scent you could add some essential oil drops of your preferred choice. Just mix them together with the other oils that you've used.

CBD Infused Edible Foods

For those of you who enjoy cooking and perhaps want to get a bit creative with your food this could be something for you. When discussing the method of extracting CBD oil from the cannabis plant, it was mentioned you will be able to infuse the oil in coconut oil, olive oil or butter. CBD-infused butter or oil will enable the CBD to be ingested. Something you can remember, and it's quite simple, is that anytime you want to use some CBD in your food it will be present in the oils or butter you have infused with the CBD. You can use the oils in salads or other cooking, the same as the butter. Use those to prepare your recipes and you will be injecting the CBD without even knowing it. For example, you can make CBD infused cookies. See below. This recipe will make approximately 18 cookies.

Ingredients
- 1 cup of sugar
- 2 ½ cups flour, (and some extra for rolling)
- 1 tsp. baking powder
- 1 cup of CBD-infused coconut oil or butter
- 1 egg
- 1 tsp. salt
- 1 tsp. vanilla

Optional: You could use powdered sugar and some milk if you want to make frosting.

If you would like your cookies to be less CDB potent just change a portion of the CBD infused butter then replace it with standard butter. You can choose how much you would like to substitute.

Cooking Process:
1. Beat the CBD-infused coconut oil or butter, vanilla, egg, and sugar in a bowl (large) and use a mixer on a

medium speed to ensure all the ingredients are combined thoroughly.

2. Using another bowl, mix all the dry ingredients together.

3. Add the dry ingredients to the CBD-infused butter. Do this a bit at a time, and stir while you are doing this until all the ingredients have been incorporated.

4. You will now have a dough mixture, which you must cover and then refrigerate for at least one hour or a little longer.

5. Take the dough out of the fridge and preheat the oven to 375°F or 180°C.

6. Roll the dough on a flat surface that has been generously floured making it approximately ⅓ inch thick.

7. Cut the cookies using a cup or mug upside down. Press out perfect circles and then transfer them to an ungreased baking sheet. You could use cookie cutters of all different shapes and sizes if you like. It's up to you, but just remember that if the cutters are larger than a cup there will probably be less than 18 cookies.

8. Bake them in the oven for about 10 or 12 minutes or until the cookies are a light golden color.

9. Remove tray from the oven and transfer the cookies to a cooling rack letting them completely cool before you frost them (if this is what you will do).
Frosting - Combine some powdered sugar with some milk and stir until you have the desired consistency. Next, add the food coloring as desired.

RESEARCH PAPERS ON CANNABIS AND ITS MEDICINAL BENEFITS

Below is a list of some research papers on cannabis and its medicinal benefits. There are many more and you can do your own research if you so choose.

-Consroe P and Wolkin A. Cannabidiol--antiepileptic drug comparisons and interactions in experimentally induced seizures in rats. J Pharmacol Exp Ther. 1977 - Apr;2011

-Jones et al. Cannabidiol exerts anti-convulsant effects in animal models of temporal lobe and partial seizures. Seizure. 2012.

-Borgelt et al. The pharmacologic and clinical effects of medical cannabis. Pharmacotherapy 2013.

-Gloss and Vickrey B. Cannabinoids for epilepsy. Cochrane Database 2014.

-Iuvone et al.Neuroprotective effect of cannabidiol, a non-psychoactive component from Cannabis sativa, on beta-amyloid-induced toxicity in PC12 cells. J Neurochem. 2004

- McAllister et al. The Antitumor Activity of Plant-Derived Non-Psychoactive Cannabinoids. J Neuroimmune Pharmacol. 2015

THANKS FOR READING

We really hope you enjoyed this book. If you found this material helpful feel free to share it with friends. You can also help others find it by leaving a review where you purchased the book. Your feedback will help us continue to write books you love.

The Smart Reads library is growing by the day! Make sure and check out the other wonderful books in our catalog. We would love to hear which books are your favorite.

Visit:

www.smartreads.co/freebooks

to receive Smart Reads books for FREE

Check us out on Instagram:

www.instagram.com/smart_readers

@smart_readers

Don't forget your 2 FREE audiobooks.
Use this link www.audibletrial.com/Travis to claim
your 2 FREE Books.

SMART READS ORIGINS

Smart Reads was born out of the desire to find the best information fast without having to wade through the sheer volume of fluff available online. Smart Reads combs through massive amounts of knowledge compiles the best into quick to read books on a variety of subjects.

We consider ourselves Smart Readers, not dummies. We know reading is smart. We're self taught. We like to learn a TON about a WIDE variety of topics. We have developed a love for books and we find intelligence attractive.

We found that each new topic we tried to learn about started with the challenge of finding the pieces of the puzzle that mattered most. It becomes a treasure hunt rather than an education.

Smart Reads wants to find the best of the best information for you. To condense it into a package that you can consume in an hour or less. So you can read more books about more topics in less time.

OUR MISSION

Smart Reads aims to accelerate the availability of useful information and will publish a high quality book on every major topic on amazon.

Smart Reads hopes to remove barriers to sharing by taking the copyright off everything we publish and donating it to the public domain. We hope other publishers and authors will follow our example.

Our goal is to donate $1,000,000 or more by 2020 to build over 2,000 schools by giving 5% of our net profit to Pencils of Promise.

We want to restore forests around the globe by planting a tree for every 10 physical books we sell and hope to plant over 100,000 trees by 2020.

Doesn't it feel good knowing that by educating yourself you are helping the world be a better place? We think so too...

Thanks for helping us help the world. You Smart Reader you...

Travis and the Smart Reads Team

WHY I STARTED SMART READS

Every time I wanted to learn about something new I'd have to buy 20 books on the topic and spend way too long sorting through them and reading them all until I arrived at the big picture. Until I had enough perspectives to know who was just guessing, who was uninformed and who had stumbled upon something remarkable.

I wished someone else could just go in and figure that out for me and tell me what matters. That's how smart reads was born. I want smart reads to be a company that does all that research up front. Sorts through all the content that is available on each topic and pulls out the most up to date complete understanding, then have people smarter than me package the best wisdom in an easy to understand way in the least amount of words possible.

For example, I got a new puppy so I wanted to learn about dog training. I bought 14 different books about dog training and by the time I got through the first 5 and finally started getting the big picture on the best way to train my puppy she had grown up into a dog.

Yeah she's well behaved. She doesn't poop in the house. I can get her to sit and come when I call. But what if someone else went in and read all those books for me, found the underlying themes and picked out the best information that would give me the big picture and get me right to the point. And I'd only have to read one book instead of 15.

That would be amazing. I would save time. And maybe my dog would be rolling over, cleaning up after my kids and doing the dishes by now. That my friend, is the reason I started smart reads. Because I wanted a company I can trust to deliver me the best information in an easy to understand way that I can digest in under an hour. Because dog training is one of many subjects I want to master.

The quicker I can learn a wide variety of topics the sooner that information can begin playing a role in shaping my future. And none of us knows how long that future will be. So why not do everything we can to make the best of it and consume a ton of knowledge. And I figured all the better if I can also make a positive difference in the world.

That's why we're also building schools, planting trees and challenging ideas about copyright's place in today's world. Because as a company we have to be doing everything we can to support the ecosystem that gives us all these beautiful places to read our books. Thanks for reading.

Travis

Customers Who Bought This Customers Who Bought This Book Also Bought

Mint As Medicine: Discover The Powerful Healing Properties of Herb in Treating Headaches, Allergies, Asthma, Clarity and Peace of Mind

The Powerful Benefits of Myrrh: Effective Myrrh Recipes For Healthy & Beauty, Oil Pulling Therapy, Creativity, Aromatherapy and Improving The Mind

Beginner Gardening: Growing Vegetables and Ornamentals

Eating Clean: Detox, Reduce Weight, Fight Inflammation and Reset Your Body

Natural Ways of Boosting Testosterone: How to
Bulk Up and Put Your Sex Drive in Overdrive

Epsom Salt_Holistic Recipes for Beautiful Skin,
Pain Relief and Relaxation

Dealing With Anxiety: Modern Techniques for an
Age Old Condition

Probiotic Dieting: The Miracle of Probiotics in
Healing Your Gut, Trimming Belly Fat and Weight
Loss